9 months of wonder

a monthly guide and journal prompts
for the conscious mother-to-be

rachel garahan

Published by Familius LLC, www.familius.com

PO Box 1249, Reedley, CA 93654

Familius books are available at special discounts for bulk purchases, whether for sales promotions or for family or corporate use. For more information, contact Familius Sales at orders@familius.com.

Library of Congress Control Number: 2023943380

Print ISBN 9781641709965

EPUB ISBN 9781641708623

Kindle 9781641708616

Fixed PDF 9781641708609

Printed in China

Cover illustration by Aislinn Hanley

Interior and back cover illustrations by Maria Schoettler

Edited by Lindsay Sandberg, Shaelyn Topolovec, and Brooke Jorden

Cover and book design by Rachel Garahan and Brooke Jorden

10 9 8 7 6 5 4 3 2 1

First Edition

9 months of wonder

a monthly guide and journal prompts
for the conscious mother-to-be

rachel garahan

for mothers and the

children who made us

May you be blessed with quiet confidence

That destiny will guide you and mind you.

May the emerging spirit of your child

Imbibe encouragement and joy

From the continuous music of your heart,

So that it can grow with ease,

Expectant of wonder and welcome.

JOHN O'DONOHUE, "FOR A MOTHER-TO-BE"

introduction

"Giving birth and being born brings us into the essence of creation, where the human spirit is courageous and bold and the body, a miracle of wisdom."

HARRIETTE HARTIGAN

For each woman who finds herself walking on the path of motherhood, the journey toward birth is a sacred rite of passage. Like all great journeys, it's one we embark on with no certain outcome, the path unfolding before us with each step that we take.

I write this as I pass my own pregnancy years with three young children in tow, each having brought their own gifts, trials, and thresholds to cross inside myself upon their arrivals. Just as I was a different woman and mother with each of my babies, you, too, will grow and change in ways you can't imagine. Being a mother is the ultimate mirror, healer, and teacher; pregnancy is just the first of many experiences in receiving these offerings.

This is a time like no other, a season of limbo: the baby is here but not here. We ourselves enter a dreamy phase between being and becoming, suspended in wonder with amazement at what we are creating and curiosity for who we are carrying.

How paradoxical for pregnancy to be referred to as "expecting." We can never know what it will be like on the other side, and in truth, *we're not supposed to.* The books we read, the advice we seek, the things we buy, the plans we make, the promises we make for things we'll do or never do—all in an effort to control a situation that is, by nature, unknowable.

We can get so caught up in the new life growing within us—distracted with facts and logistics, shoulds and shouldn'ts—that we might easily forget to acknowledge the other transformation taking place as well: the redefining of our own identity. Sometimes, the realization of our evolving self is abrupt and jarring; other times, it's so gradual that we don't notice how much we've changed until months or years later. Whether this is your first, second, third child, or more, each baby marks the transition between the woman you were and the woman you will be.

9 Months of Wonder is designed to help you to document the liminal space between here and there while softening into the season you're in. In these pages, you'll find a safe place to record and process your experiences, reflect on the ups and downs, move through fears, and honor the metamorphosis taking place in you as you give birth to the new life of your child and new parts of yourself.

Educating and preparing is a good thing. Planning is a beautiful part of the process. But if this journal can offer anything, it's to serve as a continual reminder to be inquisitive, loosen your grip, and leave room for the magic of the unimaginable—this is a journey worth being surprised for.

This book uses the terms "mother" and "woman" for consistency, to recognize the gift and power of the female body for its ability to give birth, and to honor the maternal line that has carried us through the ages.

However, I recognize that not all birthing people identify with these names. This journal is intended to serve as a space of respite and reflection for anyone on their journey through pregnancy, and as a support for their partners as well. If these identifiers are not ones that resonate, please substitute with ones that do.

BLISS LIST

01 /   Lean in to a slower rhythm

02 /   Get back to basics with a healthy diet and natural
       home + beauty products

03 /   Increase protein to ease nausea and fatigue

04 /   Keep up with existing movement rituals and routines

05 /   Rest when your body asks you to

06 /   Begin a good novel

07 /   Find a midwife or doctor you resonate with

burrow

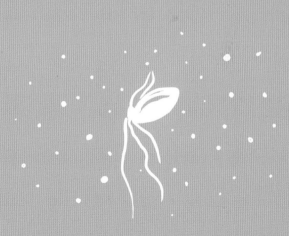

"The mothers who remind us, no matter who we are, that our first country was a woman's body, and our first element was water, and that our first reality was darkness."

MEGGAN WATTERSON

In these earliest weeks of pregnancy, you carry a secret that maybe only you, and perhaps your partner surmise. It's a delicate time when the egg that will become your child makes its way to the womb and finds a place to nestle. Before a solid bond is established between your body and your seedling of a baby, it's important to rest and allow this new life to take root.

The first trimester is when symptoms may be the most extreme— ironically, as this is also typically when no one yet knows you're pregnant. Even with your partner, it may be hard to convey how different you feel or communicate your changing needs when, outwardly, you appear the same as you always have.

But speaking up for your needs is your first exercise in caring for two. For you are the Mother-well: a precious source of life-giving energy, both as the foundation for your family and quite literally as your child's lifeline in the womb. Exercising your advocacy muscle will take you far in parenthood, and right now, creating a safe, strong container will serve you both. So when responsibility commands that you go about life as usual, protect your energy and allow yourself permission to say when the day is done. Put your feet up, read books, eat well, stay hydrated, and rest.

This is not to say that being busy is overall a bad thing—women have been working through pregnancies since the beginning of time. We are strong beings who can handle more than we think, and keeping occupied is healthy for both the body and mind. Most anything you did comfortably before, you can safely continue doing; the goal is to find balance in staying active without pushing your limit.

Of course, this may be easier said than done. When there is always something to do, maintaining boundaries or prioritizing our own needs can be hard. In general, Western culture tends to demand so much focus on work and productivity that it can feel difficult to honor personal needs at *any* point in our lives. But if there's a perfect time to practice putting ourselves first, the short season of pregnancy is it.

In the first trimester, nausea and exhaustion serve to slow us down for a reason. During this time, see if you can surrender and let yourself be just where you are. If frustration or resistance around "not doing enough" arise, try setting your thinking mind aside and tuning in to what is true for you today without comparing it to how you operated before. It's okay to lean in to the temporary place that is now. You'll be back on your feet soon enough.

The consistent theme you'll find throughout this journal is listening to your own quiet knowing—and then actually honoring what you know to be true. So when you feel called to rest, lean in to it. Even if you can't pull back completely, slow movements and calm breath have a grounding effect that go a long way. When in doubt, keep it simple. Our biggest pressures most often come from within.

a picture of us . . .
with each month, we grow

invite

(weeks 1–4)

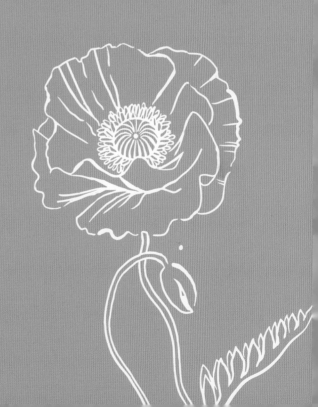

*"(here is the root of the root and the bud of the bud
and the sky of the sky of a tree called life; which grows
higher than soul can hope or mind can hide)
and this is the wonder that's keeping the stars apart
i carry your heart (i carry it in my heart)"*

E. E. CUMMINGS

I n this first month, you may not know yet if you are pregnant. Maybe you're setting the intention to become pregnant, oscillating between thinking you are or aren't, or juggling many conflicting feelings. Before it's known for sure, you are in a space of uncertainty, occupying a place on both sides of the threshold.

Is your baby still a longing? A whisper? A presence that you feel or have already confirmed? Wherever you are, use the opportunity to connect energetically with them now. It is never too early to send them love or share your honest feelings.

If the idea of emotionally investing in the life inside of you so early on is overwhelming, that's completely understandable. We each have our own levels of comfort here, and while there is benefit to saying yes to a journey, whatever it may bring, honor what's right for you.

Depending on how you feel, you might like to invite your baby into your world, walking them through your home and introducing them to the space where they will grow and play. You could talk to them about any plans you may have, about the future you envision, or guide them through each part of your day as though their mind's eye is perched on your shoulder.

By using the power of intention to help strengthen your energetic connection, these practices can serve as an invitation, welcoming your baby in.

But before we get too far ahead, it's helpful to look at where you are and from where you've come. Where does this season in life find you?

While this journey is nothing short of magic, with it comes a transformation and a sense of loss of your former self. Whether it's the you-before-children or the you-when-it-was-just-you-and-your-older-children that you mourn, every transition comes with complicated feelings.

As you step into your new, expanded iteration, know that the "old you" doesn't actually go anywhere. At your core, you still are, and always will be, you. But the process of bringing another life into your family—from pregnancy through the first year or longer—is a journey that will take you apart and rearrange you; at some points in the middle, it may seem as though you've lost some of your pieces. The journaling prompts in this chapter serve to remind you both of who you are today and what you're experiencing now, a trail of breadcrumbs helping you find your way back to all the parts of yourself.

this month . . .

Ways I connect with you	
Things I say to you	The energy you bring
Celebrating the life inside of me	
Getting ready for you by	Special things bought or received
You seem to like it when . . .	

Ways I care for myself	
Feelings	Sensations
In my mind . . . themes, mantras, and affirmations	
Dreams	Intuitions
How I'm evolving . . . body, closet, lifestyle, and the everyday	

EMBRACING THE EXPERIENCE

Cravings + Aversions		
Nervousness or Confidence	Hopes or Fears	
Joy, Reverence + Awe		
Surprises	Changes	
Complaints, Confessions, Heartaches, Challenges		

THE JOURNEY OF DISCOVERY

Learning, reading, listening to . . .		
How I connect with my partner	Focuses this month	
Where I feel most loved and supported		
Advice	Reactions	
Looking forward to . . .		

Three words to describe pregnancy right now:

_____

_____

This month in your life (a story to share or things to remember):

_____

_____

_____

_____

_____

_____

_____

_____

_____

_____

_____

_____

_____

What led you to this point, and how do you feel now that you're here? Did you always want a baby, or did the desire come more recently? Was the conception journey difficult or easy? Take time to reflect on the unique path that brought you here, along with all the thoughts and feelings that come with it.

Consider how your understanding of pregnancy and birth has been shaped by the media and entertainment, cultural messaging, or your own personal experiences thus far. How might these combined influences be affecting your current expectations?

_____

_____

_____

_____

_____

_____

Describe an average day in your current life:

_____

_____

_____

_____

_____

_____

_____

What makes you, you? For example, what are you known for? What's your favorite trait about yourself? What do you value most?

_____

_____

_____

_____

_____

_____

_____

What is your favorite part about your life right now? What makes you feel strong and fully alive? Who do you love to be around?

_____

_____

_____

_____

_____

_____

_____

What brings you energy and lights you up just thinking about it?
How do you connect to your creativity? When do you feel in flow?

_____

_____

_____

_____

_____

_____

What other ambitions do you have? Where else are you putting
your energy besides motherhood?

_____

_____

_____

_____

_____

_____

_____

_____

What dreams or fears do you have about how this pregnancy will transform you?

_____

_____

_____

_____

_____

_____

_____

_____

_____

_____

_____

_____

_____

_____

_____

_____

_____

_____

a picture of us . . .

with each month, we grow

open

(weeks 5–8)

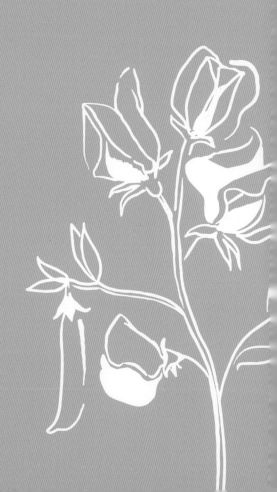

"We must be willing to get rid of the life we've planned, so as to have the life that is waiting for us."
JOSEPH CAMPBELL

This month, you may hear your baby's heartbeat for the first time. If it wasn't real before, it is now—and, if your partner is able to be with you for the experience, this is often the moment that it feels real for them, too. There is a new life pulsing inside of you, ready for nurturing and reverence.

With your due date in mind, you may already be counting down for all that needs to be done before then. Just remember—pregnancy is a short, unique, and concentrated season of life. How do you truly wish to spend it?

Before planning your to-do list, consider focusing these early weeks on setting intentions for the things you can control, like your mindset and supporting actions. These intentions will not only serve as attainable goals, but also as a foundation to support all else that is out of your control.

For example, as part of the major spiritual transformation that pregnancy is, it's common for social dynamics to shift during this time or for issues with friends or family to arise (whether openly or privately). If this is true for you, trust it's all an opportunity for growth.

Or, you may notice a common theme arising throughout many areas of your life over the next several months. If so, it can be helpful to note the type of situations that are showing up and acknowledge the particular energy this pregnancy brings.

Layered in with our personal experience is our environment too—the time and place in which we exist. My second pregnancy was marked by California wildfires and mudslides; my third marked by COVID. We live in an uncertain world—the best we can do is practice acceptance and openness amidst it, and pregnancy is no exception.

Whatever is happening, whether in your world or the world at large, consider any challenges as part of a rite of passage. We each walk through the fire in our own way during our initiation into motherhood. If you aren't able to have the "perfect" pregnancy, remember this is all part of your baby's and your story. By surrendering our ideals, we can better embrace our ordeals.

this month . . .

Ways I connect with you	
Things I say to you	The energy you bring
Celebrating the life inside of me	
Getting ready for you by	Special things bought or received
You seem to like it when . . .	

Ways I care for myself	
Feelings	Sensations
In my mind . . . themes, mantras, and affirmations	
Dreams	Intuitions
How I'm evolving . . . body, closet, lifestyle, and the everyday	

EMBRACING THE EXPERIENCE

Cravings + Aversions	
Nervousness or Confidence	Hopes or Fears
Joy, Reverence + Awe	
Surprises	Changes
Complaints, Confessions, Heartaches, Challenges	

THE JOURNEY OF DISCOVERY

Learning, reading, listening to . . .	
How I connect with my partner	Focuses this month
Where I feel most loved and supported	
Advice	Reactions
Looking forward to . . .	

Three words to describe pregnancy right now:

_____

_____

This month in your life (a story to share or things to remember):

_____

_____

_____

_____

_____

_____

_____

_____

_____

_____

_____

_____

_____

What is most important as you search for a midwife or doctor? Do you feel more comfortable with an intuitive approach or a medical one?

What are some guiding words for how you want this pregnancy to feel?

_____

_____

_____

_____

_____

What does well-being mean to you? How can you incorporate just a little more of it into your daily life?

_____

_____

_____

_____

_____

_____

_____

_____

What are some activities that feel restful? Consider three ways you can create more spaciousness in your everyday.

When you look back, what will you wish you had done during this time?

First hints that you were pregnant and the day you knew you definitely were:

Who you told first and how you told your partner:

a picture of us . . .

with each month, we grow

align

(weeks 9–12)

"Ground . . . it is what holds and supports us . . . a place on which to stand and a place from which to step."

DAVID WHYTE

You began this journey privately and spent the first trimester getting used to the idea of your expanded identity as a mother and protector. Before you begin to outwardly show or share with the world at large, take this time to set a solid foundation in place with your partner.

Note: Throughout this journal you will find references and prompts geared specifically towards your partner. If you are a single parent, your "partner" may be a friend or family member you can lean on. If you don't have support readily available or you're simply not comfortable with letting others in, know you are deserving of care and support in whatever form you choose.

For many couples, it's the mother who handles the majority of choices surrounding a baby registry, shower, and birth planning. However, getting your partner involved in the decision-making process early is a good way to help them feel included and valued.

We can become so focused on pregnancy and our baby, we might forget that as a new parent, even more significant than the relationship we have with our new child is the one we have with our partner. Making aligned choices with them now will not only help you both to build confidence amidst the sea of conflicting information but unite you in a feeling of togetherness as you set the tone for parenthood.

In the day-to-day, moms often take on the brunt of childcare responsibilities, whether the result of culturally-expected gender roles or habits established from the physical realities of pregnancy, birth, and breastfeeding. But this can lead to resentment, burnout, or both as time goes on. The more you can include your partner from the beginning, the more capable and confident they will feel to support you in shared caretaking responsibilities once the baby has arrived.

And remember, just as they are your primary support person, you are also theirs. Your partner may be feeling anxious or overwhelmed and not know how to voice it; getting in the habit of talking openly about how you're both feeling is a good place to start. Making sure they have the space for restful time alone, therapy sessions, a night out, a weekend away with their friends, or the opportunity to be acknowledged in a way that resonates are all ways you can support them.

While it may be hard to verbalize needs in the moment, think about how each of you could best feel best supported, and find a time to share your thoughts. The questions in this chapter can help to guide your conversation.

ways your partner could support you

- *Listening without trying to fix*
- *Preparing your favorite breakfast or beverage*
- *Taking care of house chores*
- *Exercising or adopting healthy lifestyle changes together*
- *Doing the bedtime routine with older children*
- *Running you a bath*
- *Arranging your pillows at night*
- *Offering no-strings-attached massages (lots!)*
- *Connecting through the journey together: turn appointments into lunch dates, look at a baby app together before bed, share a parenting book that resonated, and give them plenty of opportunities to talk to baby and feel them move.*

43

this month . . .

Ways I connect with you	
Things I say to you	The energy you bring
Celebrating the life inside of me	
Getting ready for you by	Special things bought or received
You seem to like it when . . .	

Ways I care for myself	
Feelings	Sensations
In my mind . . . themes, mantras, and affirmations	
Dreams	Intuitions
How I'm evolving . . . body, closet, lifestyle, and the everyday	

EMBRACING THE EXPERIENCE

Cravings + Aversions	
Nervousness or Confidence	Hopes or Fears
Joy, Reverence + Awe	
Surprises	Changes
Complaints, Confessions, Heartaches, Challenges	

THE JOURNEY OF DISCOVERY

Learning, reading, listening to . . .	
How I connect with my partner	Focuses this month
Where I feel most loved and supported	
Advice	Reactions
Looking forward to . . .	

Three words to describe pregnancy right now:

_____

_____

This month in your life (a story to share or things to remember):

_____

_____

_____

_____

_____

_____

_____

_____

_____

_____

_____

_____

If you have a partner, how are they adjusting to pregnancy? What seems to engage them most in preparations?

_____

_____

_____

_____

_____

_____

_____

_____

_____

_____

Who is your primary support person? Who else in your circle can you rely on?

_____

_____

_____

_____

_____

What feelings, concerns, goals, or decisions do you want to share with your partner? What questions do you have for them?

_____

_____

_____

_____

_____

What things can you do to support each other right now? Once the baby arrives?

_____

_____

_____

_____

_____

_____

_____

_____

What are your respective birth plan preferences? While there's time to figure out the specifics, is there anything that either of you have strong or definite feelings about?

_____

_____

_____

_____

_____

When you have conflicting preferences or expectations, what are some ways you and your partner come back together?

_____

_____

_____

_____

_____

_____

_____

_____

When sharing your choices with your family and friends, are there topics you are open or not open to receiving advice on? Together, how can you establish healthy boundaries to protect your decisions and your partnership?

_____

_____

_____

_____

_____

_____

_____

_____

_____

_____

_____

_____

_____

_____

_____

What are your hopes for your partnership during the pregnancy?
What do you imagine it will look like after delivery?

_____

_____

_____

_____

_____

_____

_____

_____

_____

_____

_____

_____

_____

_____

_____

_____

_____

_____

BLISS LIST

01 /   Find a movement class you love

02 /   Join a pregnancy or mother's group, either in person
or online

03 /   Upgrade to comfortable maternity clothing or add a
few new items you feel good in

04 /   Savor the awe of feeling baby's first flutters

05 /   Honor this time as a rite of passage

06 /   Stay anchored in the sea of outside opinion

bloom

"Belong to love. Bless,
Join, fashion the deep forces,
Asserting your nature, priceless and feminine.
Peace, daughter. Find your true kin."

GENEVIEVE TAGGARD

As you enter into your second trimester, this typically easeful stage of pregnancy is one in which symptoms subside, energy rises, your baby bump emerges, and the worry of the first trimester tends to blossom into excitement for all the discoveries to come.

This can be a lovely time, and one to savor. From a sensory perspective, you'll begin to feel the first flutter of movements and kicks while your baby responds to your touch, tastes the flavors of the foods you eat, and hears the sounds of your life. The dog barking, street sounds, siblings' and parents' voices—this muted melody is the background of their world, one which will feel comforting and familiar once they arrive. Through your shared perceptions, your inner and outer experiences are becoming interwoven.

The second trimester is all about expansion. As your body grows to make space for two, you can begin to make space in your life as well by preparing the baby's area, sharing the news, building a community, going on adventures, and beginning to think about what type of baby celebration you may want to have. *(See Chapter 8 for more specific ideas.)*

Let the expansion of this time flow through to your spiritual and emotional space as well. The chapters in this section will help you to heal your past, sink into the present, and dream about the future.

a picture of us . . .

with each month, we grow

connect

(weeks 13–16)

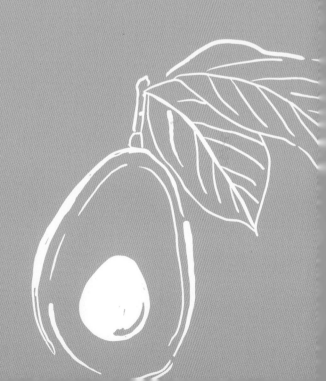

"The circles of women around us weave invisible nets of love that carry us when we're weak and sing with us when we're strong."

SUSAN ARIEL RAINBOW KENNEDY

In many Eastern traditions, it's believed that in the first three months of pregnancy, the baby's soul drifts between the physical and ethereal plane; not until the fourth month does its soul formally merge with its physical body. This aligns with Western thought, which sees the fourth month as a time when a more secure connection between the baby and the mother's body is established and the risk of loss drops significantly. In both perspectives, passing into week thirteen marks the end of the most vulnerable stage of pregnancy.

This is a time when many feel confident enough to announce that they're expecting. While it's often a joyous one, as you share your news, you become susceptible to everyone's varied advice, input, and observations, whether you want them or not.

You've already set a foundation and discussed boundaries with your partner. Now is also a good time to remind each other that while others may share their strong opinions, the ones that matter most are your own. That said, who else's advice you respect and value?

As a parent, having a supportive community that aligns with your values can make all the difference in your experience. Your circle may be made up of family members, friends, caregivers, parent groups, specialists, experts, or other mothers you follow online. And while each serves a valuable role, this section focuses on the particular gift of mom friends with similar due dates—and eventually, a child of the same age as yours.

With the somewhat predictable arc of new motherhood—up in the middle of the night, issues with feeding and digestion, not feeling like yourself, being always available while also, strangely, never available—there is much to be said for confiding in another mother who is right in the thick of it with you, or recently has been.

When things are difficult or overwhelming (or you're just wanting to keep your family healthy) it's natural to isolate at home. This can be one of the most challenging aspects of having a new baby, and a time when many mothers experience varying levels of anxiety about not doing enough or not doing things the "right" way.

Support yourself by finding a moms' group (either in person or online) or choosing even just one other person you resonate with deeply; this community or person may become your lifeline in the early months.

Whether through yoga studios, women's circles, community organizations, educational centers, or social media platforms, try out different options until you find one group—or even just one mom—that's right for you.

And in any situation, don't be afraid to speak your truth, even if you're the first to share or if your experience feels different than what others seem to be going through. Not only will your message likely resonate in ways you didn't expect, but it's the best way to forge authentic connections.

Whether one-on-one or in a group setting, there is tremendous power in being able to show up as ourselves and be accepted exactly as we are.

suggestions for responding to outside opinion

When it comes to outside input, respond in a way that doesn't give away your personal power. If it's coming from a stranger or someone you won't see again, you might say something non-committal like, "Good idea, I'll think about that."

If it's someone you're in regular communication with, you might say something firmer like, "Thanks for the input, but we've already decided on a [birthing location, name, stroller] we feel good about."

If you find repeated unsolicited advice coming from the same person, don't be afraid to be direct and say something like, "I appreciate your support, but I'm really not interested in advice."

Regardless of what comes your way or how you respond, you can always envision a filter that allows you to hold on to any helpful pieces that resonate while letting the rest pass through.

this month . . .

Ways I connect with you	
Things I say to you	The energy you bring
Celebrating the life inside of me	
Getting ready for you by	Special things bought or received
You seem to like it when . . .	

Ways I care for myself	
Feelings	Sensations
In my mind . . . themes, mantras, and affirmations	
Dreams	Intuitions
How I'm evolving . . . body, closet, lifestyle, and the everyday	

EMBRACING THE EXPERIENCE

Cravings + Aversions	
Nervousness or Confidence	Hopes or Fears
Joy, Reverence + Awe	
Surprises	Changes
Complaints, Confessions, Heartaches, Challenges	

THE JOURNEY OF DISCOVERY

Learning, reading, listening to . . .	
How I connect with my partner	Focuses this month
Where I feel most loved and supported	
Advice	Reactions
Looking forward to . . .	

Three words to describe pregnancy right now:

_____

_____

This month in your life (a story to share or things to remember):

_____

_____

_____

_____

_____

_____

_____

_____

_____

_____

_____

_____

First flutters and feeling your baby move:

_____

_____

_____

_____

_____

_____

_____

_____

Plans and feelings on finding out (or waiting to know) your baby's sex:

_____

_____

_____

_____

_____

_____

_____

Who you've shared with, or how you plan to share the news with others (or not):

_____

_____

_____

_____

_____

_____

What does your social life look like right now? Are you someone who likes to be with others often, or are you more comfortable with lots of alone time?

_____

_____

_____

_____

_____

_____

_____

_____

_____

How comfortable are you with vulnerability and sharing with others? Are you open to forming new friendships at this time?

_____

_____

_____

_____

_____

_____

_____

_____

Which people are most supportive in your life? Who do you consider your inner circle?

_____

_____

_____

_____

_____

_____

_____

Whose opinions do you trust? Do you know any aligned mom friends who you can count on as resources? Who do you look up to as a mother or in the parenting expert world?

What are you seeking most out of community? Do you know of any local mom groups in your area? Do a bit of research and list some options that you feel could be a good fit or worth checking out, either in-person or online.

a picture of us . . .
with each month, we grow

dream

(weeks 17–20)

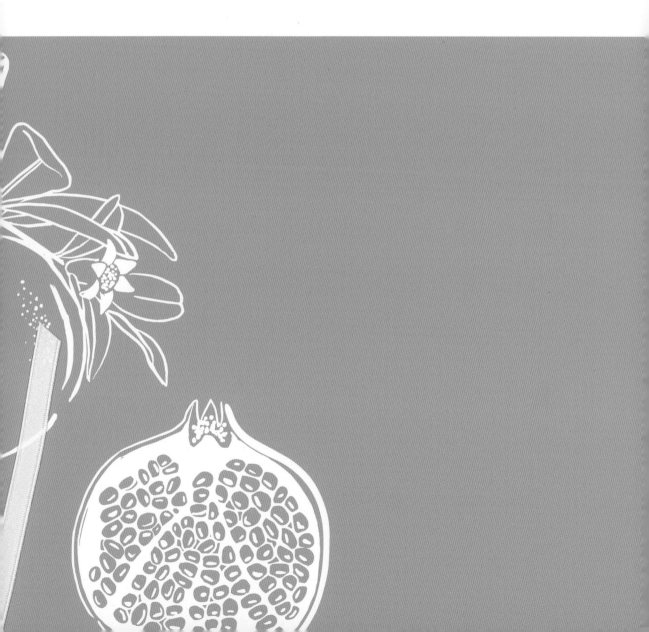

"Do not ask your children
to strive for extraordinary lives. . . .
Make the ordinary come alive for them.
The extraordinary will take care of itself."

WILLIAM MARTIN

In the fifth month, you may get to see—not just imagine—your baby's face in an ultrasound and decide whether or not to find out their sex. For some parents who choose to have an anatomy scan, this may be a joyous time of relief or confirmation. For others, it may reveal new gender or genetic information, disrupting the bond they'd been building with their baby and the future they'd been envisioning. If you are adjusting to the idea of something new, know that any reactions or feelings you may have are perfectly okay.

While staying in the present helps to maintain a healthy mindset, envisioning who your baby will be, what your family might be like, and who you will become can bring great joy. As the creator of your family, imagining goes hand in hand with intention and the process of conscious creation.

That said, life is a great dance with the universe; we are always co-creating with it. And part of its magic is that it includes all that is beyond our imagination.

The prompts in this chapter offer space to record the hopes and dreams you hold for your family at this moment in time.

embracing the unexpected

- SURRENDER | What relief might be found in releasing the struggle to control? Often, our most difficult or dissapointing moments ultimately offer peace as they help us realize we were never really in control in the first place. To surrender is not to give up, it's to give *over*. To acknowledge the gift of greater forces at play; to accept that we don't need to understand everything, and to trust that there is more to our path than we currently can see.

- GRATITUDE | When we're stuck in a pattern of negative, judgmental, or victim-based thinking, gratitude is a mindfulness practice we can use to shift from focusing on all that isn't going well to all that is. No matter how small or insignificant acknowledgments of gratitude may seem, this practice of actively receiving each moment uncaps a bubbling wellspring of insight that can build momentum to carry us forward.

- OPENNESS | Try allowing yourself to observe your situation with curiosity. What is it here to teach or share with you? By remaining open to possibility, you may discover it's a redirection offering something you didn't know you needed.

- ONENESS | Take some time to stop to really observe nature. When we do this, it's undeniable how giving, perfectly synchronized, and self-supporting it is. Everything needed for it to thrive is inextricably a part of it. Don't forget that you too are a part of nature, a pattern woven into the greater design of life. By tapping into its inherent abundance, you can know that what is needed is always present.

- ALLOWING WHAT IS | Each of us experiences suffering at some point in our lives; it's part of the human experience. When challenging feelings arise, know that you are allowed to feel exactly as you do, without anything to change or fix. Emotions are simply energy in motion—let them wash over you and through you. By acknowledging them rather than ignoring or pushing through them, you create the spaciousness to process them in real time. Be soft with yourself.

73

this month . . .

Ways I connect with you	
Things I say to you	The energy you bring
Celebrating the life inside of me	
Getting ready for you by	Special things bought or received
You seem to like it when . . .	

Ways I care for myself	
Feelings	Sensations
In my mind . . . themes, mantras, and affirmations	
Dreams	Intuitions
How I'm evolving . . . body, closet, lifestyle, and the everyday	

EMBRACING THE EXPERIENCE

Cravings + Aversions	
Nervousness or Confidence / Hopes or Fears	
Joy, Reverence + Awe	
Surprises / Changes	
Complaints, Confessions, Heartaches, Challenges	

THE JOURNEY OF DISCOVERY

Learning, reading, listening to . . .	
How I connect with my partner / Focuses this month	
Where I feel most loved and supported	
Advice / Reactions	
Looking forward to . . .	

Three words to describe pregnancy right now:

_____

_____

This month in your life (a story to share or things to remember):

_____

_____

_____

_____

_____

_____

_____

_____

_____

_____

_____

_____

What are your aspirations outside of motherhood? How does your baby fit into the larger vision you have for your own life's goals?

_____

_____

_____

_____

_____

_____

_____

_____

_____

_____

_____

_____

How do you envision yourself as a mother? What are some keywords that embody the kind of mother you hope to become?

_____

_____

_____

_____

_____

It is said that children grow in the garden of their parents' relationship. Consider your own relationship with your partner—what kind of space are you creating? What example do you want to model?

_____

_____

_____

_____

_____

_____

_____

_____

What does parenting mean to you? Describe the kind of relationship you'd like to have with your kids:

_____

_____

_____

_____

_____

_____

_____

What kind of family do you hope to have? What do you do together? How do you connect?

_____

_____

_____

_____

_____

_____

_____

_____

_____

_____

What types of memories do you want to build? Which traditions from your own families do you want to carry over? What new traditions might you want to create?

_____

_____

_____

_____

_____

_____

What sort of people do you want your kids to be as they grow into adults? What future do you envision for them? What values do you want to instill?

_____

_____

_____

_____

_____

_____

_____

What expectations are you holding on to? What are they protecting you from? How will you feel if things don't turn out the way you plan?

envisioning your baby:

I found out your biological sex | I didn't find out. My hunch:

_____

Characteristics I hope you get from me/ your other parent:

_____

_____

_____

In my mind, I envision you to look like this:

_____

_____

Traits I hope you posess:

_____

_____

Right now, we call you . . .

_____

_____

The types of names we like for you (traditional, unique, nature-based, family names, etc):

_____

_____

_____

Your (other parent/ grandparent/ sibling/ _____)
likes these names:

_____

_____

_____

First names we like:

_____

_____

_____

_____

_____

Middle names we like:

_____

_____

10. My dreams for you . . .

a picture of us . . .

with each month, we grow

empower

(weeks 21–24)

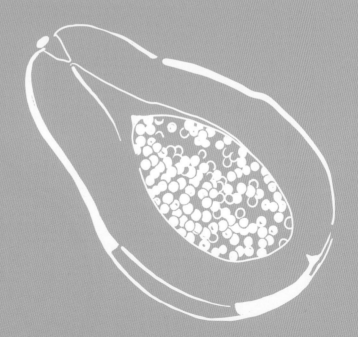

"If you listen to [your children], somehow you are able to free yourself from baggage and vanity and all sorts of things, and deliver a better self, one that you like. The person that was in me that I liked best was the one my children seemed to want."

TONI MORRISON

In the sixth month of pregnancy, change is happening at a rapid pace, for both you and your baby—and as you transition into your third trimester, your body is no doubt looking and feeling different from before. A phase often marked by weariness and impatience, let this time of physical growth lead the way for personal growth.

It has been said that motherhood reveals a woman's roughest edges, and the same is true for pregnancy. Before your baby arrives, you are still mostly just you, making it a good time to work on unresolved issues in order to integrate new learnings and show up as best you can for your child once they arrive.

Through the study of epigenetics—an emerging science that looks at how mindset, behavior, and environment affect genes—we are beginning to learn the amazing power a pregnant woman has on three generations at once: herself, her unborn child, and her unborn grandchild, through the impression her life makes on the eggs in her womb. Not only does this offer insight into the power we hold for the future, but into the impact of the past as well: all the stories and experiences our maternal grandmother carried while pregnant had an effect on our mother and on us. With this knowledge, we can recognize the magnificent potential our bodies hold for evolution, and choose to utilize it for positive change.

This month, allow your attention to be focused on transforming judgment and composting it into compassion through forgiveness.

This can be done by looking closely at the way we judge ourselves and others, by forgiving those who came before us and did the best they could with the circumstances, resources, and knowledge they had, and by choosing to forgive our past, current, and future selves for the many mistakes we have made or will make as imperfect beings.

By acknowledging this layered and continual process, we can start to accept and heal our own unhelpful patterns and thoughts so we don't pass them on to the next generation. If we can learn to do this for ourselves, we will empower our children with the loving capacity to do the same, passing the positive shift forward.

meditating through fear

Whether inherited or learned, a result of past experience or the unknown, impending motherhood can inspire some of our greatest fears. Though uncomfortable, allowing ourselves to sit with them can bring us back to a place of empowerment. If you notice fears arising, try this meditation for spaciousness and ease:

Find a quiet place to sit without distractions. Focus on your breathing and allow yourself to witness what comes up. Name the fear that comes to mind. Where do you feel it in your physical body? Continue to focus on your breathing and allow your fear to take shape. Envision all of the details. What happens, and what happens after that? Explore the full cycle of what this fear means to you by walking through each scenario, considering your reactions and next steps until you reach a place of knowing that whatever comes, there's a way you can move through it. By giving space to your fears rather than pushing them away, you help them to loosen their grip on you.

Note: If you have a history of trauma, mental health issues, or feel overwhelmed by your fear, please consult your doctor or therapist for individualized support.

this month . . .

Ways I connect with you	
Things I say to you	The energy you bring
Celebrating the life inside of me	
Getting ready for you by	Special things bought or received
You seem to like it when . . .	

Ways I care for myself	
Feelings	Sensations
In my mind . . . themes, mantras, and affirmations	
Dreams	Intuitions
How I'm evolving . . . body, closet, lifestyle, and the everyday	

EMBRACING THE EXPERIENCE

Cravings + Aversions	
Nervousness or Confidence	Hopes or Fears
Joy, Reverence + Awe	
Surprises	Changes
Complaints, Confessions, Heartaches, Challenges	

THE JOURNEY OF DISCOVERY

Learning, reading, listening to . . .	
How I connect with my partner	Focuses this month
Where I feel most loved and supported	
Advice	Reactions
Looking forward to . . .	

Three words to describe pregnancy right now:

_____

_____

This month in your life (a story to share or things to remember):

_____

_____

_____

_____

_____

_____

_____

_____

_____

_____

_____

_____

_____

_____

How are you feeling in your pregnant body? Are you enjoying your changing shape? Describe how this physical evolution has felt for you.

_____

_____

_____

_____

_____

_____

Name any unhealthy attachments, judgments, or negative thoughts about your physical body, personality, or capabilities. What can you let go of that no longer serves you?

_____

_____

_____

_____

_____

_____

_____

Consider for a moment the possibility that your child's soul might have consciously chosen you. Which of your gifts, challenges, and life experiences make you their imperfectly perfect mom?

_____

_____

_____

_____

_____

_____

_____

_____

_____

_____

_____

_____

_____

_____

_____

_____

_____

The Mother Line: What was your mother like? What stories or history do you know from her life or lineage?

What do you know about your birth and what you were like as a baby? If there are any emotional wounds surfacing at this time, how can you nurture and support your inner child?

_____

_____

_____

_____

_____

_____

_____

_____

_____

_____

_____

_____

_____

_____

_____

_____

_____

_____

What patterns, feelings or thoughts have you noticed coming up for you? How might these be viewed as opportunities for growth?

_____

_____

_____

_____

_____

_____

_____

_____

_____

_____

_____

_____

_____

_____

_____

_____

_____

What qualities do you admire or judge in other moms or your own? What makes a "good" mom? What makes a "bad" mom? Where do you think these ideas originated?

_____

_____

_____

_____

_____

_____

_____

_____

_____

_____

_____

_____

_____

_____

_____

_____

Consider what your parent/child relationship could look like if you choose to hold onto limited, negative, or outdated thinking. How might things be different if some of these thoughts or beliefs were released?

_____

_____

_____

_____

_____

_____

_____

_____

_____

_____

_____

_____

_____

_____

_____

_____

BLISS LIST

01 /   Make or save playlists to listen to during labor
       and delivery

02 /   Empower yourself with birth stories, podcasts,
       and documentaries

03 /   Deepen your meditation or mindfulness practice

04 /   Keep your hands and mind busy with a project
       or craft

05 /   Take a day off and pamper yourself or let others
       nurture you

06 /   Appreciate, admire, and honor your beautiful, life-
       giving body

nest

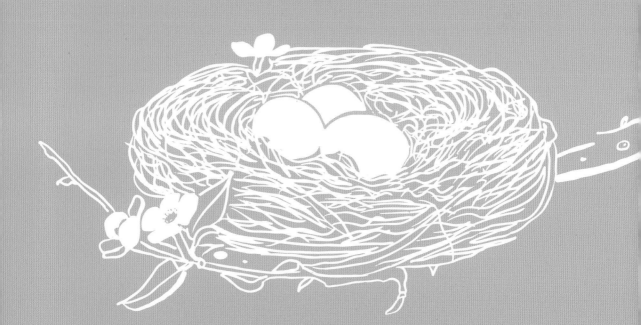

"Stillness is what creates love. Movement is what creates life. To be still and still moving—that is everything."

DO HYUN CHOE

In the final months of pregnancy, ease into the rhythm of a slower beating drum. With your body heavy and time moving slow as honey, there is a sweetness to savoring these last months with you and your baby as one.

Just like in the first trimester, it can be challenging to feel both called to slow down and anxious about doing so. To keep the calendar flexible while continuing to make plans. To desire fully focusing on the coming of your baby while desperate for distractions from the wait.

Trying to trust the process while trying to control it—this is a time of contradiction, and that's okay. The best you can do is continue to move forward with the next best step, while honoring the place you are in.

Through the ages, one way mothers-to-be have prepared for this sacred transition is by nurture from other women in their community. Today, the tradition continues in varied forms, often in the form of a party or celebration. It can be fulfilling to be witnessed in full bloom and fun to be showered with support, wisdom, gifts, and love. Yet some feel uncomfortable in the spotlight or aren't interested in accumulating more things.

While there's no rule that says you must be celebrated, whether in a small group or extended to a wider circle, consider the idea of being recognized in your own way as the capable, powerful, and life-giving woman that you are.

Another way to honor this time is to plan a maternity photo shoot. Professionally taken or captured by a friend, in nature or at home, alone or with your family, photographs are a beautiful way to remember this moment in life and the radiance of your pregnant belly. Even if you don't feel your best or can't imagine wanting photos of yourself at this point, you might be surprised looking back on them later and cherish this special time.

As you reach closer towards birth, this final trimester is also a good time to get more specific about your intentions here. Giving birth is one of the most empowering journeys a woman can ever make—but depending on how respected and supported she feels during this experience, it can be just as easily disempowering.

This section will help you to consider how you want to create your experience.

a picture of us . . .

with each month, we grow

gather
(weeks 25–28)

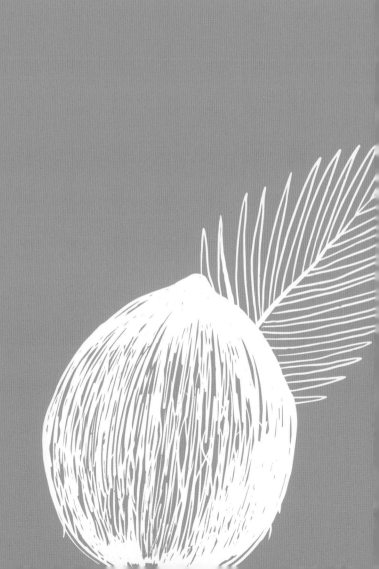

"Every baby comes with a loaf of bread under his arm."
OLD SPANISH SAYING

By the seventh month, you've fully transitioned to the third trimester, where time seems to somehow both slow down and speed to the finish line. There is still so much to do, yet at the same time, it may feel like your little one can't come soon enough.

In these moments, if your heart is longing to know your sweet baby's face but your brain keeps thinking about the endless list of things to complete before they arrive, if you're feeling anxious about costs and logistics or how this new, tiny being will fit into an already full life, may you find comfort in the time-honored mantra *Babies Bring Abundance*.

Across varied Eastern traditions, it's believed that all creation energy is sourced from the same energetic center within. Meaning that inspiration, fertility, and prosperity are bounties that run together, fed from the same spring. So while it's normal to feel overwhelmed by the unknowns, let this be a reminder of the supportive abundance already flowing for you.

During this time, addressing the things you *can* control helps to offer structure and ease the mind. Making preparations is a natural extension of excitement, and so things like establishing birth intentions or setting up a nursery, or getting other details organized can be uplifting while clearing mental space, allowing more bandwidth for anything else that may arise.

Whether gathering information and goods, preparing your physical space, or planning for those more practical and predictable elements in the birth and the postpartum period, in this chapter, you'll find questions and considerations to support you through the process of organization.

postpartum details

Although by this point "pregnancy brain" has no doubt set in, this is a great time to have important conversations with your employer, colleagues, and other primary support people about your postpartum schedule so everyone is clear on your plan. Doing so helps to ensure a smooth transition and puts in place the boundaries and support you need to avoid being distracted and overwhelmed later on.

With your partner, do your best to leave no decision-making stone unturned now before newborn sleep deprivation sets in later. Choose a time when you're both feeling calm and relaxed and look through the questions at the end of this chapter together. Write down your preliminary thoughts, considering this a first draft in a conversation that can continually evolve.

When it comes to daily life, consider all your current responsibilities and how you might ease them during the postpartum time. This could include advance food preparation (researching recipes, preparing freezer meals, or looking into meal delivery options) dog walking, cleaning, baby care, care for older children, postpartum doula support, or scheduling dates for any out-of-town visitors.

Although there are certainly things you *could* take care of on your own during postpartum, try to give your future self the gift of rest during this unique and special time, as much as circumstance allows.

nesting

Whether your baby will have a room of their own or a special nook, take care of any decorating now, while your energy is still relatively high. Have your partner support you with the "heavy lifting" jobs like painting, wallpapering, putting up shelves, or assembling furniture. Seeing things come together will help you feel that much closer to and ready for baby's arrival, and doing it together is a fun way to share in the anticipation.

birth words

While there's no script for exactly how things are going to go during the birth, you can provide your partner with a list of supportive things to say. Save notes from birthing books you may be reading or advice from parenting classes, and keep track of visualizations and phrases you find inspiring. During intense moments, many partners find security in having a list of these approved, go-to encouraging reminders and are glad to know how to be there for you in a way that's most comforting and effective.

birth logistics

There will be more specific questions relating to birth intentions in Chapter 10, but at this point, it's helpful to go over some of the less emotional aspects. If you plan to deliver outside of the home, schedule a tour so you know where to park, if you'll need cash for parking, where to enter from, where to sign in, etc. During the tour, you'll get to see the type of room you'll be in, which can help you better envision your experience. You can also begin to plan the route to the hospital and scope out places nearby (restaurants, hotels, etc.) in case you need resources.

If you're delivering at home, look into the supplies needed and consider how and what your setup will be.

hospital birth considerations

If you're planning on a hospital delivery, many choices will need to be made in the 24 hours after birth. Spending the time to understand all of your options in advance will give you the opportunity to research and decide what feels best for you. In the exhaustion and bliss of bringing your child into the world, there will be interruptions in the form of wellness checks and medical staff coming and going from your room. Discussing these things ahead of time with your partner and birth team will allow them to best support and advocate for you, or even speak on your behalf if you're resting.

While hospital staff and specialists can guide you and offer expertise, keep in mind that you are in charge, most things are not required, and you are allowed to question or decline anything you don't feel comfortable with. Many hospitals will be happy to accommodate low-intervention births in whatever way that means to you. Just be sure to make decisions from an informed place, and remember that the most important factor is having a safe delivery experience for both you and your baby.

Continue the previous months' conversations and get more specific with your partner by discussing the topics below.

topics for discussion

- *PICC line / IV*
- *Labor induction*
- *Epidural*
- *Skin-to-skin bonding*
- *Delayed cord clamping*
- *Cord blood banking*
- *Placenta saving*
- *Vaginal swabbing (postcesarean)*
- *Nursing*
- *Bonding time*
- *Hep B vaccine*
- *Vitamin K*
- *PKU*
- *Eye antibiotic*
- *Circumcision*
- *Pacifiers*

postpartum partner support

Make a list of ways your partner can help after the baby is born. Most partners are more than happy to pitch in, as long as they know how. Carrying the baby in the front pack, washing bottles, or preparing meals and snacks for you both are examples of ways they could be supportive.

It's okay not to know your exact needs right now; this is a space to simply brainstorm and gather ideas, adding to the list when new ones arise. Then use this list for easy reference after delivery to make the postpartum period smoother.

-
-
-
-
-
-
-
-
-
-

this month . . .

Ways I connect with you	
Things I say to you	The energy you bring
Celebrating the life inside of me	
Getting ready for you by	Special things bought or received
You seem to like it when . . .	

Ways I care for myself	
Feelings	Sensations
In my mind . . . themes, mantras, and affirmations	
Dreams	Intuitions
How I'm evolving . . . body, closet, lifestyle, and the everyday	

EMBRACING THE EXPERIENCE

Cravings + Aversions	
Nervousness or Confidence	Hopes or Fears
Joy, Reverence + Awe	
Surprises	Changes
Complaints, Confessions, Heartaches, Challenges	

THE JOURNEY OF DISCOVERY

Learning, reading, listening to . . .	
How I connect with my partner	Focuses this month
Where I feel most loved and supported	
Advice	Reactions
Looking forward to . . .	

Three words to describe pregnancy right now:

_____

_____

This month in your life (a story to share or things to remember):

_____

_____

_____

_____

_____

_____

_____

_____

_____

_____

_____

_____

_____

Describe your baby's special place in the home. What are you envisioning for it? What have you gathered so far, and what still needs to be done?

_____

_____

_____

_____

_____

_____

Where will you be delivering the baby? Are there any logistics can you organize for the birth now?

_____

_____

_____

_____

_____

_____

_____

_____

What are your shared expectations around childcare and parenting duties? How will you divide things like diaper changes, feeding, nighttime or weekend care, sleep training, etc.? How can you best communicate as partners when one person needs to tap out?

_____

_____

_____

_____

_____

_____

_____

_____

_____

_____

_____

_____

How are you currently financially supporting your family? Will this change once the baby is here? What is your work transition plan?

_____

_____

_____

_____

Do you believe you deserve a restful postpartum period? If you are able to take maternity leave, how much time will you take and what is your intention for how you want to spend it? Whatever your situation, what are some ways you can build in extra support during this time?

_____

_____

_____

_____

_____

_____

_____

Consider your daily responsibilities, both at home and in other areas of your life. Where can you delegate in order to begin clearing things off your plate?

_____

_____

_____

_____

_____

_____

_____

_____

_____

_____

_____

_____

_____

_____

_____

_____

How do you feel about postbirth visitors and guests? Are there any guidelines/timelines you'd like to set or specific types of support you'd like to request?

During the no-sex healing phase after birth, what other forms of intimacy can help keep you connected?

a picture of us . . .

with each month, we grow

receive

(weeks 29–32)

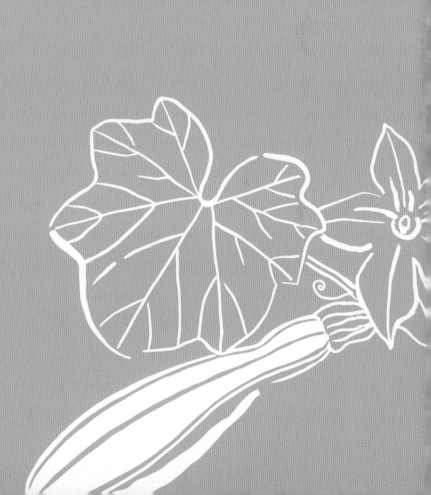

"Our elders say that ceremonies and rituals are the way we 'remember to remember.'"

ROBIN WALL KIMMERER

Before you retreat inward in your final weeks, the eighth month is a wonderful time to be acknowledged by others, honoring the huge shift that's taking place in yourself and your life.

For millennia around the world, cultures have held ceremonies to recognize this exceptional rite of passage; to prepare, fortify, and bless new mothers for birth and beyond. Over time, the ancient practice has shifted from one that is mother focused to one that focuses primarily on the baby and gift giving. This is a wonderful way to gather important items and be surrounded by love and support.

However, if you are interested in an experience that speaks more to the sacred transition of birth and new motherhood, you may consider having or incorporating elements of what's known as a *Mother Blessing*. Originating from the Navajo Blessingway ceremony for mothers-to-be, this tradition focuses solely on nurturing them with loving care.

A modern interpretation of this intentional gathering could be in addition to a traditional baby shower, with a large group or small one, with just one friend, in person or virtually, or even by yourself (a spa day, massage, or pedicure certainly counts as loving care). In whatever style you choose, the important thing is allowing yourself the opportunity to be honored in a way that feels good to you.

mother blessing inclusions to consider

- Sit in a circle (to represent a container of support) while sharing encouragement, blessings, prayers, stories of birth and motherhood, and words of acknowledgment. Guests can bring a poem, song, passage from a book, or simply share from the heart.

- Share food together in celebration— catered, hosted, or pot-luck style.

- Make a bracelet or necklace from beads brought by each guest for you to wear or keep near you during labor.

- Weave a flower crown from flowers brought by each guest for you to wear and then save as a dried keepsake.

- Gift each guest with a small candle to light in their own homes once they hear the birth is underway as a way of holding space for you.

- Let friends create a special mother throne adorned with flowers or ribbons, pampering you with shoulder, foot, and hand massages or an herbal foot bath and scrub.

- Hold a thread ceremony in which a spool of red thread is passed around the circle of women, each guest looping it around her wrist before passing it to the next person as an act of support and connectivity. Once the woven circle is complete, everyone takes turns cutting the strings off the person beside them, tying a piece around their wrist. Each guest then winds up wearing a string bracelet that they keep on as a reminder of you until they hear that birth is underway. At this point, they each cut their bracelet to symbolize supporting you in energetically releasing your baby while sending blessings and prayers.

- Create a gift basket of books, journals, lotions, sprays, crystals, oils, favorite beauty products, herbs, chocolates, and other special just-for-mom gifts.

- Tie-dye onesies. While not specifically mother focused, it's an activity that's always fun and will fill your little one's drawers with a sweet reminder of your closest circle of friends.

a note on registries

Gifts are a beautiful way to be celebrated, supported, and prepared, but know this: you don't need to buy into the commercialized version of motherhood that tells you all the things you should have in order to be the "right kind" of mom.

Soft and structured baby carriers, a quality stroller, and a good rocking chair were my best and longest-lasting investments. As for other items, many of the things I couldn't live without for one child had no relevance for the others. The moral of the story being that while we may hope *being fully equipped* will help with *feeling fully equipped*, the items you're considering are for an unknown future and a tiny person whose preferences you don't yet know! Keep it simple.

That said, when creating a registry, what things make you smile when envisioning your little one wearing or using them? There is always room for joy.

Last of all, don't be afraid to register for a few non-baby-related pleasures. These can make all the difference in the postpartum days, whether by making your life easier or by helping you to feel "together"—especially when you're feeling anything but.

mom's wish list

- Face + body masks, scrubs, balms, or lotions

- Bath soaks and sitz bath blends

- Favorite candles, incense, or diffusers

- Eye mask

- Nursing-friendly pajamas

- Cozy socks or blankets

- A good book

- Mom bag or backpack

- Large water bottle

- Ceramic mug or bowl

- Postpartum tea blends

- Superfoods, protein powders, or other nourishing pantry goods

- Massage or manicure/pedicure gift certificates

- Meal train contribution or restaurant gift certificates

- Gift certificates for convenient online shopping

- Gift certificates for house cleaning

this month . . .

Ways I connect with you	
Things I say to you	The energy you bring
Celebrating the life inside of me	
Getting ready for you by	Special things bought or received
You seem to like it when . . .	

Ways I care for myself	
Feelings	Sensations
In my mind . . . themes, mantras, and affirmations	
Dreams	Intuitions
How I'm evolving . . . body, closet, lifestyle, and the everyday	

EMBRACING THE EXPERIENCE

Cravings + Aversions	
Nervousness or Confidence / Hopes or Fears	
Joy, Reverence + Awe	
Surprises / Changes	
Complaints, Confessions, Heartaches, Challenges	

THE JOURNEY OF DISCOVERY

Learning, reading, listening to . . .	
How I connect with my partner / Focuses this month	
Where I feel most loved and supported	
Advice / Reactions	
Looking forward to . . .	

Three words to describe pregnancy right now:

_____

_____

This month in your life (a story to share or things to remember):

_____

_____

_____

_____

_____

_____

_____

_____

_____

_____

_____

_____

_____

How comfortable are you with receiving, whether it be attention or things?

_____

_____

_____

_____

_____

What does *nurture* mean to you? What would make you feel relaxed and cared for? Allow yourself to dream and brainstorm here, without limits or judgments or "shoulds":

_____

_____

_____

_____

_____

_____

_____

_____

_____

_____

What ways might you like to be celebrated? Is there anyone you can ask to help create this?

_____

_____

_____

_____

_____

_____

When it comes to baby items, consider the ones that are most important to you. Which do you want to gather in advance and which can you wait on?

_____

_____

_____

_____

_____

_____

_____

When it comes to preparing your baby's space, do you have colors or nursery themes that appeal to you or materials you like? What about items or types of things you'd like to limit in the home?

As you've grown throughout your pregnancy, what changes do you notice in the way you see yourself? In how you relate to others?

_____

_____

_____

_____

_____

Consider anything you want to accomplish or enjoy in the last weeks before your due date. Where do you need closure before motherhood? Finish this sentence: "Before my baby arrives, I'd like to . . . "

_____

_____

_____

_____

_____

_____

_____

_____

List all the things you are grateful for in your pregnancy and currently in your life:

a picture of us . . .
with each month, we grow

anticipate

(weeks 33–36)

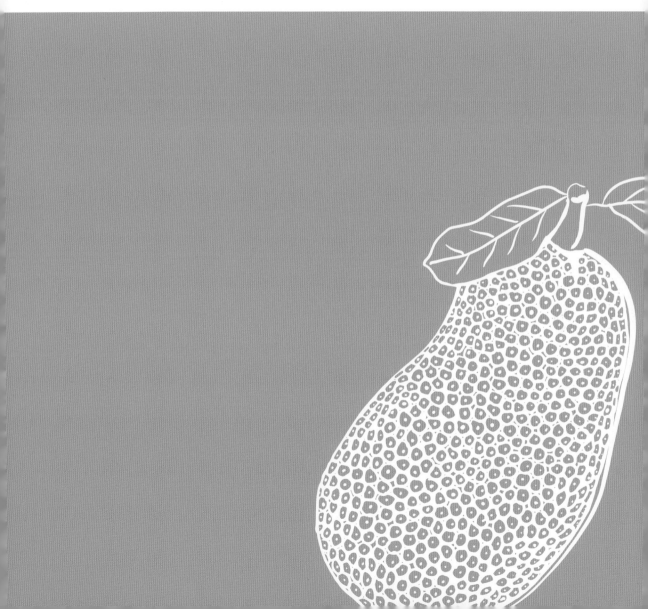

"Whenever and however you give birth, your experience will impact your emotions, your mind, your body, and your spirit for the rest of your life."

INA MAY GASKIN

In the ninth month, you may be desperate to know your sweet baby's face, craving ultrasound images, feeling physically uncomfortable, or anxious to have your body back. However, just as in birth, this discomfort is temporary, and although there may be a feeling of just wanting to "get through it," you can apply the same lessons regarding impatience to both scenarios.

As you prepare for labor and beyond, try not to let this time fly by, distracted by things that don't ultimately matter. Rather than letting your to-do list deplete you, do things that will fill your cup and infuse you with energy to carry you through the postpartum days. Visit with friends. Enjoy moments of peace alone or with your partner at your favorite places. Engage in activities that bring you joy and connect you to the childlike enjoyment of play.

Each time a woman goes through the experience of childbirth, it's as though a reset button has been pressed on life. Babies have a way of making us realize just what is important—everything else falling away by necessity. So use the prompts in this section to write down everything on your mind: questions, to-do's, loose ends you need to tie up; anything that will help to clear space and clarify what matters most to you.

This is also a good time to begin to bring your energy and attention inward towards your ideal birthing experience.

From *early labor* (which can last anywhere from a few hours to a few days, and typically feels mild enough that you can carry on with your normal activities) to *active labor* (the phase in which you are focusing all of energy and attention on birthing) focusing on the specifics surrounding your birth intentions can help you feel as present and prepared as possible.

Part of this includes reviewing your preferences and desires with your partner if you haven't already *(see page 110)*, discussing all the options together so that you both feel aligned and fully informed.

Whether home or hospital, cesarean or vaginal, medicated or unmedicated, induced or not, remember that birth is inherently natural and there is no "right" way about it.

Any way your baby is born has the potential to be your own empowered choice—whether planned in advance or through intentional surrender to circumstance. If you notice feelings of hesitation, disappointment, or concern surrounding your decisions thus far, consider what specifically is bothering you, along with any elements you might be able to improve, adjust, or come to terms with in order to bring more peace before delivery.

this month . . .

Ways I connect with you	
Things I say to you	The energy you bring
Celebrating the life inside of me	
Getting ready for you by	Special things bought or received
You seem to like it when . . .	

Ways I care for myself	
Feelings	Sensations
In my mind . . . themes, mantras, and affirmations	
Dreams	Intuitions
How I'm evolving . . . body, closet, lifestyle, and the everyday	

EMBRACING THE EXPERIENCE

Cravings + Aversions	
Nervousness or Confidence	Hopes or Fears
Joy, Reverence + Awe	
Surprises	Changes
Complaints, Confessions, Heartaches, Challenges	

THE JOURNEY OF DISCOVERY

Learning, reading, listening to . . .	
How I connect with my partner	Focuses this month
Where I feel most loved and supported	
Advice	Reactions
Looking forward to . . .	

Three words to describe pregnancy right now:

_____

_____

This month in your life (a story to share or things to remember):

_____

_____

_____

_____

_____

_____

_____

_____

_____

_____

_____

_____

_____

_____

How does it feel to begin moving things off your plate? Is any part of you having trouble letting go? List all of the things still weighing on your mind, outstanding to-do list items, or loose ends that need to be tied up. Organize them into priorities.

Looking at your list from above, what are the things that ultimately don't matter? Delegate them or decide to let them go.

If you could share anything with your baby, what would you want
to tell them?

envisioning your ideal labor and birth scenario, part 1

Envision the twenty-four hours before you go into labor. How will you spend that day?

_____

_____

_____

_____

When does labor ideally begin and where are you when that happens? How do you spend early labor?

_____

_____

_____

_____

What's your idea of the perfect last meal to have before or during early labor?

_____

_____

_____

_____

What can your partner do while you are in early labor (time contractions, be with you, pack the car, feed pets, etc.)?

_____

_____

_____

_____

If you are not giving birth at home, what can your partner do while you settle in to your space (set up things like playlists, a fan, a birth altar, bedside items, a phone charger , etc.)? If giving birth at home, how else can your partner help?

_____

_____

_____

_____

If you had your choice, would you prefer active labor to be slow and steady or fast and intense? Invite this experience in.

_____

_____

_____

_____

_____

Who is with you in the room during active labor, and what are their roles? Are there any parameters you'd like to communicate?

_____

_____

_____

_____

What about phones and communication during labor for your partner or others in the room? Are there any boundaries you'd like to set into place here?

_____

_____

_____

_____

How do you imagine active labor to feel? What elements support you (candles, pictures, foods/beverages, playlists, meditations, totems, jewelry, people)?

_____

_____

_____

_____

How well do you cope with pain? What can you do to mentally or physically work through the pain with greater ease?

_____

_____

_____

_____

What do you plan to visualize during pushing? Are there any reminders that could help you stay focused on this? List any specific words or phrases that would be helpful for you to hear from your partner or birth team during active labor.

_____

_____

_____

_____

Baby and Mama set the mood. What is your guiding word for the energy you'd like to contribute to this experience?

_____

_____

_____

_____

How do you spend the first moments/hours together after your baby is born? Describe anything you would like to happen or not to happen:

_____

_____

_____

_____

What is your first meal postbirth? Will you rely on what the hospital offers, or will it be something you can bring with you, order in, or have your partner pick up nearby?

_____

_____

_____

_____

How long do you wait before sharing the news with others and how do you do so (individual texts or calls, group texts, or connecting with a point person who shares the news with a defined group of people)? Are there boundaries you'd like to communicate with your inner circle surrounding sharing details about the baby (news of arrival, name, sex, photo) on social media or with others?

_____

_____

_____

_____

envisioning your ideal labor and birth scenario, part 2

Now that you have a complete birth vision, *let it all go*. All preferences aside, remember that the main goal is to bring your baby safely into your arms. Try to release all expectations and stay open to whatever is needed in the moment, rolling with whatever happens and feeling empowered by knowing you're making your best possible choices along the way.

Things will inevitably go differently than planned, whether in a big or small way. Letting go of our birth ideals is just one of many tests of selflessness we encounter on our path as a mother. Can you set aside your own plans and desires in order to allow what is best for your baby?

By acknowledging that babies are active participants in the birth process, we can more easily surrender to the fact that, sometimes, they're born the way they need to be instead of the way we want them to be, and it's all a part of their own unique story.

a picture of us . . .
with each month, we grow

surrender

(weeks 37–40+)

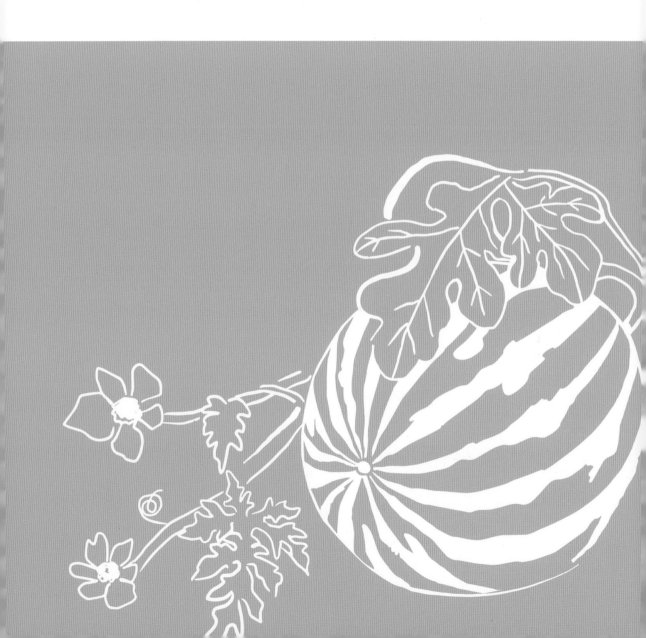

"We think we are the captain of the ship. . . . [But] when you go into labor, you see that you are not the captain of the ship. You are the ship. There is no captain. There are only waves."

KAREN MAEZEN MILLER

Just as crops yield at a general time in the season, the estimated arrival of your baby is not a perfect science, so try not to fixate on your exact due date. Babies come in their own time and in their own way. Whether early, late, or just as predicted, their birth-day will be right on time.

As you approach the end of your pregnancy and your body begins to physically prepare for labor, an energetic portal opens in you as well. Mothers being the channel through which children are brought into this world, it's a time when many say "the veil" said to separate spiritual worlds "feels thin." Here, you may find yourself in an extra dreamy state, your mind cotton fluff as your focus naturally turns more and more inward.

In these final days, stay close to home and give yourself permission to let go of any final details that didn't get done, focusing on purposeful or easeful ways to pass the time depending on what you're feeling drawn to do.

While some will want or need to take it easy, not everything needs to be restful. A burst of drive and stamina is often a sign that you are near, and especially during this time, it can be helpful to direct that strong energy to wherever your intuition calls. Remember, you are the Mother-well—whatever you need to do in order to feel good in your mind and body, your baby will benefit from too.

If there comes a time when you do feel completely ready for your baby's arrival (whether or not every box is checked and preparation is made) tune in and let them know.

Just as you energetically invited them in during the first four weeks, you can energetically open the door for them again. Of course, doing so doesn't guarantee they'll join you right away, but remember that you are co-creating this journey together; in connection every step of the way.

ways to pass the time

- *Finalize baby's area*

- *Wash the baby clothes*

- *Build out your mama nest (the space in your home where you and your baby will spend much of your time in your first weeks)*

- *Take long walks, naps, baths, and calls with friends*

- *Clean or organize the house*

- *Lean in to whatever inspires you, even if it seems like an unreasonable last-minute project*

- *Batch prep freezer meals and postpartum snacks*

153

preparing for childbirth

Trust your body; trust your baby. This is a good mantra for all of pregnancy, but especially now. As women, we *know* how to birth babies—yet of all the mammals on earth, we are the only ones to allow ego to interfere, leading us to question our ability.

However your labor and birth unfolds, stay in the moment, anchored in your intentions to support whatever your baby needs or your inner voice is asking of you. Give yourself permission to go inward, undistracted by the external and uninhibited in your actions—getting your thinking brain out of the way helps to tap into your instinctual, primal knowledge. You are allowed to take up space; you are allowed to take your time. Delivering in a way that makes you feel safe and supported is fundamental to a easeful and empowered birth.

a birthing bag for the senses

There is no "ultimate" birthing bag checklist. Each experience varies tremendously, even for the same mother between different births. No matter what you end up packing in yours, consider these sensory inclusions to calm and ground you in your birthing space.

- **See:** *ultrasound images, photos, art, totems, or anything else that makes you feel you feel supported, powerful, inspired, relaxed, or expansive.*

- **Feel:** *cozy blankets, loose and comfy clothes, bathrobes, socks, favorite balms or oils, jewelry*

- **Hear:** *playlists, meditations, headphones*

- **Taste:** *simple whole-food snacks, hydrating beverages*

- **Smell:** *favorite lotions, essential oil diffuser, essential oils (peppermint to energize and lavender to calm)*

preparing for postpartum

In the first weeks after birth, you and baby will spend much of your time resting and recovering. Begin to prepare your cozy nest with this postpartum time in mind. Where in the house will you be most comfortable? Since your little one will primarily need just sleep, milk, diaper changes (and of course your loving care!) the things you'll want within easy reach will be simple and practical. A soft light, supportive pillows, diaper-changing supplies, and things for your comfort (water, snacks, balms, phone charger, or book) will all make this space a refuge.

It can be a big adjustment, going from being fully independent to having limited mobility in the early days or with a newborn on you most of the time. Set yourself up for success by stocking your kitchen with warming, gently-flavored, and easy-to-digest foods to support postpartum healing as well as any others you enjoy. Since you will be eating most of your food one-handed, consider soups, broths, smoothies, bars, cut fruit, and other things that aren't difficult to eat in bed. If you like to have things made a particular way, take the time to practice some of these recipes with your partner or support person now.

While the focus here has been primarily on you and your baby, what does your family need? Even if it's just you and your partner, they will be exhausted as well, so remember to consider meal times for your unit as a whole.

However you prepare, whether with easy-to-grab nutritious food or ready-made family meals that can be simply heated and served, having favorites on hand is an easy way to create a sense of familiarity and control, helping life run more smoothly for all.

If you have older children, they of course will need lots of support beyond just food. Meaningful gifts "from" the new baby, crafts and projects to keep them occupied, fun caregivers, and arranging playdates or activities can go a long way to meet their needs while providing you with peaceful moments to bond with your newest little one.

this month . . .

Ways I connect with you	
Things I say to you	The energy you bring
Celebrating the life inside of me	
Getting ready for you by	Special things bought or received
You seem to like it when . . .	

Ways I care for myself	
Feelings	Sensations
In my mind . . . themes, mantras, and affirmations	
Dreams	Intuitions
How I'm evolving . . . body, closet, lifestyle, and the everyday	

EMBRACING THE EXPERIENCE

Cravings + Aversions	
Nervousness or Confidence	Hopes or Fears
Joy, Reverence + Awe	
Surprises	Changes
Complaints, Confessions, Heartaches, Challenges	

THE JOURNEY OF DISCOVERY

Learning, reading, listening to . . .	
How I connect with my partner	Focuses this month
Where I feel most loved and supported	
Advice	Reactions
Looking forward to . . .	

Three words to describe pregnancy right now:

_____

_____

This month in your life (a story to share or things to remember):

_____

_____

_____

_____

_____

_____

_____

_____

_____

_____

_____

_____

_____

_____

What expectations surrounding childbirth are you still holding on to? Where could you loosen your grip, even by a little?

_____

_____

_____

_____

_____

_____

If your ideal birth doesn't go as planned, what are some alternatives you could comfortably surrender to?

_____

_____

_____

_____

_____

_____

_____

_____

_____

_____

Look back at your ideal labor and birth scenario from the previous chapter. What are three words you want to embody no matter how things go? Are you and your partner aligned in this vision?

_____

_____

_____

_____

_____

_____

What and who soothes, inspires, expands, or uplifts you?

_____

_____

_____

_____

_____

_____

_____

_____

What do you want to pack in your birthing bag?

_____

_____

_____

_____

_____

_____

What daily responsibilities do you normally handle at home and how will your family be supported during postpartum?

_____

_____

_____

_____

_____

_____

_____

_____

_____

Loose ends to tie up, last work responsibilities, the last date you can spend with your partner or have space to rest . . . what do you need in these final days to feel complete?

_____

_____

_____

_____

_____

Is there anything else standing in the way of letting you fully sink into birth and postpartum?

_____

_____

_____

_____

_____

_____

_____

_____

your circle of support: who can you call on to help with . . .

Caring for pets or older children during the birth?

Sharing the news?

Organizing a meal train?

Childcare / playdates / adventures for older children during postpartum?

Cooking, washing dishes, folding laundry, running errands, and organizing?

Mother support (time to shower or rest, supportive snacks, emotional support, etc)?

Other?

BLISS LIST

01 /   Go at your own pace

02 /   Avoid looking at your phone in the middle of the night

03 /   Take a social media break, choosing presence instead

04 /   Tune into the sweetness of new baby energy

05 /   Give gentle baby massages

06 /   Make your own list of self-nourishing priorities and
check it daily

07 /   Practice doing nothing "productive" at all

08 /   Allow others to help and care for you

09 /   Lay in a hammock, on the couch, or on a blanket
under a tree with your little one on your chest

cocoon

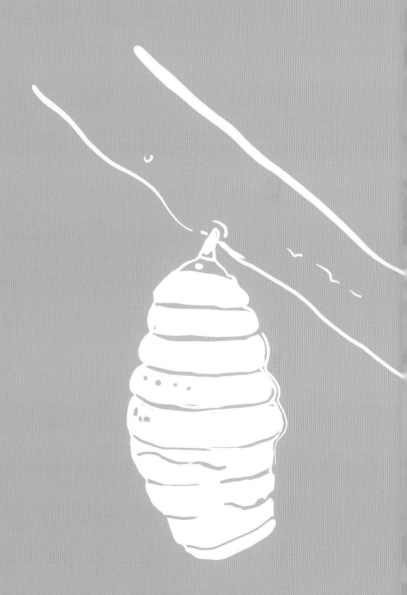

"What is required energetically at birth—expansiveness, transcendence, and openness—is quite different from what is required of women postpartum—presence, groundedness, steadfastness."

KIMBERLY ANN JOHNSON

This section encompasses birth and the first forty days (*Eastern mindset*) or six to twelve weeks (*Western mindset*) after birth. This time is imperative for healing and recovery, for parents and baby to bond, for the mother to nurture her body postbirth, and for the baby to settle into life outside the womb.

Within this "fourth trimester," you will journey through various phases of transition, each one serving to support you in adjusting to your new life with your baby:

In the first hours, you may experience an initial surge of euphoria, although for some mothers, it takes longer to settle in. Physical closeness with your baby (even if you're not yet feeling it emotionally) will help to secure your bond. Just as instinctual efforts serve a purpose in birth, age-old practices like breastfeeding, holding your baby skin to skin, gazing into their eyes, and talking or singing softly all serve a purpose: to increase bonding hormones and help soothe and support the transition and connection for you both. However your birthing journey unfolded, know that there will be time to process your transformation. For now, enjoy the magnificent life you've ushered into this world and allow yourself to feel pride, relief, and profound awe.

In the first days, it may feel like quite a shock to have full responsibility for this new, tiny human. This esoteric energy you've been communicating with, the mystery being you've been carrying and protecting all these months—it now has a face you can see, a name, a personality, preferences, needs, and a voice with which to share it all. Your time is no longer your own, and you are easing into a new rhythm where they are in charge.

In the first weeks, a whirlwind time when days and nights blur together, the ground may feel as if it's shifting beneath you. There will be tears of struggle, joy, exhaustion, beauty, and hilarity. Everything, and nothing, has prepared you for this new reality. Though you may feel precarious out in the world, find safety in the cocoon of your home sanctuary.

In the first months, as you settle into your new role and rhythm, enjoy the preciousness of this fleeting time and get to know your little one. There's no button to pause or rewind, so appreciate the time you are in and be patient with yourself in your new role. With every phase that passes, you'll find yourself pushing the boundaries of your comfort and expanding the breadth of your ability.

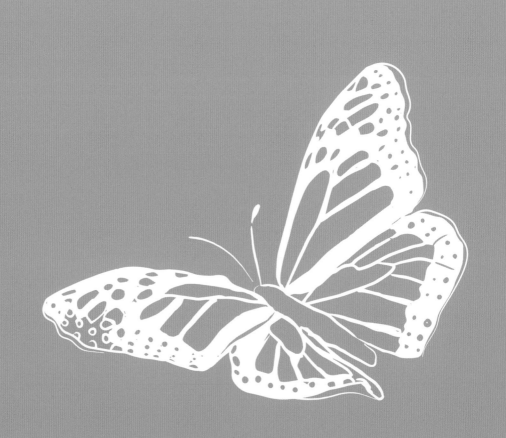

embrace

(your birth story)

"Let what you do not know come into your eyes. . . .
May your soul be at home where there are no houses."
URSULA K. LE GUIN

Dear Mother, you made it to the other side! A profound transformation has taken place in your being. You have returned full circle to where you began, yet you are not the same woman you were before.

As humans, storytelling is intrinsic to how we make sense of the world, ourselves, and our lives. Writing your birth story helps not only to integrate your own experience, but to serve as a record for your family, providing your child with the gift of connection to their own origin story.

Use this space to process, reflect on, heal from, preserve, celebrate, and honor both you and your baby's journey.

There is no perfect time to write; some may prefer to do so in the early days before the details fade while others may need time to process the events. For each mother, there will be a unique time when she feels called to write her story; it is never too late.

When you are ready, write it all—the facts and the details, the play-by-play, the unexpected, the remarkable, and the spiritual. This is your experience to share.

birth details . . .

Full name: _____

Place of birth: _____

Time of birth: _____

Weight: _____

Length: _____

Hair color: _____

Eye color: _____

Birthmarks: _____

Moon phase at time of birth: _____

Sun sign, moon sign, rising sign: _____

your birth story, in your own words . . .

Three words to describe labor + birth:

_____

_____

Who was there? What was helpful?

_____

_____

_____

_____

_____

_____

First sight of your baby:

_____

_____

_____

_____

_____

_____

The biggest surprise:

_____

_____

_____

_____

_____

What feature did you immediately fall in love with?

_____

_____

_____

_____

_____

_____

_____

_____

_____

Bliss + difficulties:

_____

_____

_____

_____

_____

First impressions of baby's energy or personality:

_____

_____

_____

_____

_____

_____

_____

What did you learn about yourself through the experience of giving birth?

_____

_____

_____

_____

_____

_____

Feelings + first impressions on motherhood:

_____

_____

_____

_____

_____

_____

_____

_____

a letter to baby . . .

a picture of us . . .
with each month, we grow

attune
(the first 12 weeks)

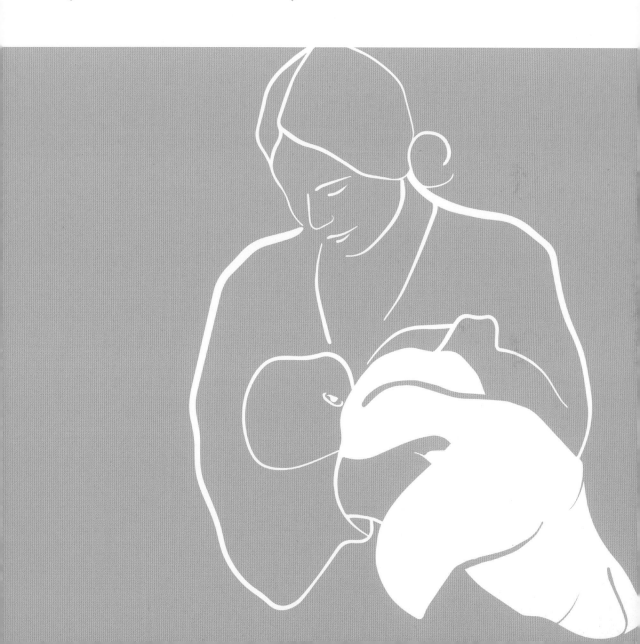

"Most parents invest endless effort and resources to ensure the best starts for their children. But mothers need a strong start too. The old ways teach us that the biggest investment is made up front. If Mom begins rested and nourished, calm and centered, she can provide the patience and sensitivity—the maternal devotion—that her baby truly deserves."

HENG OU

Although in the West it's made to seem that mothers should get back to normal as quickly as possible, the journey doesn't end at birth. This time is one for attunement—for connecting with your baby, aligning with your new rhythm, and coming full circle to reconnect with yourself.

These early months are a time of adjustment physiologically too, with immense hormone changes that play a large role in determining your moods: an initial euphoric surge to support mother-child bonding, the feeling of "baby blues" when those first blissful hormones drop, and mood swings as you navigate all the ups and downs that come with the territory of new motherhood. During this time, it can be helpful to not identify too closely with how you feel, remembering that *you* and *your emotions* are not the same.

Note: If mood swings are intense or longer lasting, know that postpartum anxiety and depression are common. If there is trauma to process or you're having trouble adjusting, seek help both professionally and from your trusted circle.

Try not to forget that immense healing is needed after birth; don't push it too soon! There is no award for who takes a walk first. Take it easy and allow others to care for you. A good practice for the early days is the 5-5-5 rule: 5 days in bed (horizontal and resting), 5 days on the bed (incorporating sitting up), and 5 days near the bed (incorporating walking around the house).

In this time, when everything is in flux, be kind to yourself. Avoid lofty or unrealistic expectations. If things feel a bit uncertain with your partner during this transition time, try to maintain open communication and emotional connection, and remember that even when things are hard, you're on the same team.

In your own routine, keeping things simple helps create a sense of structure and stability. Rely on the sanctuary of your cozy nest, focusing on soaking in the sweet new-life energy your baby brings. Being with your little one might not seem like much, but know that your loving gaze and attentive presence will serve as a foundation to nourish all of their days. You will be distracted soon enough; let them have this time with you uninterrupted.

Now is also a time to tend to yourself. If you are used to working, it may be unique to not have commitments outside of the home. How can you prioritize your own delight? Use the space below to think of the things that bring you energy or joy, and reference them often. These may be reminders to journal, listen to favorite meditations, enjoy your favorite foods, take a daily walk, or even reminders of things you don't want to do.

Newborn care can feel monotonous, and looking ahead to unstructured days can feel overwhelming. Having simple go-to rituals can provide a sense of purpose and well-being and serve as a reminder for how you want to spend this time.

Reminders for ways I can fill my own cup:

-
-
-
-
-
-
-
-
-
-
-
-

beyond the first 12 weeks

As weeks turn into months, at some point, you will look back and be shocked to learn you are no longer the parent of a newborn. After the birth of a baby, it's difficult to imagine being anything other than "new mama," but often it isn't so long before the resonance of "I am a mother" turns to hunger for more.

The first year is one of significant change and growth in this new role, and throughout it you'll discover your own inclination for selfhood. Whatever your desires, remember there is no right or wrong approach and that your relationship with parenting will evolve with each season of your life.

Yet as you slowly begin to reclaim your identity and independence, there will come the moments when you're ready to switch out the oversized clothing, get back to your pre-pregnancy routines, or take on a new project. While honoring your own timeline, know that whether through creative outlets, socialization with other adults, professional pursuits, or simply unstructured alone time, the importance of re-establishing connection to anything that brings you a sense of fulfillment and purpose *beyond motherhood* cannot be overstated.

9 Months of Wonder was created to support you through the transitional time of pregnancy and new motherhood as you expand into a new iteration of yourself. If you find yourself feeling lost, disconnected, or longing for a version of you that feels far away, look back at the entries throughout this journal as touchstones along the path that brought you here. Through these pages and your own words, may you find connection to these parts of yourself once again.

Being a mother is only one part of your identity, yet it can easily eclipse your other roles and needs if you aren't mindful about leaving space to just be *you*. Allowing the time to nourish and express all the multifaceted parts of your being will not only bring energy to your mothering journey but will help keep you connected to the woman who embarked on this path to begin with—and the one you are continually becoming.

this month . . .

Ways I connect with you	
Things I say to you	The energy you bring
My favorite times with you	
The sounds and faces you make	The items we can't live without
You seem to like it when . . .	

Ways I care for myself	
Feelings	Healing
In my mind . . . themes, mantras, and affirmations	
Dreams	Intuitions
How I'm evolving . . . body, closet, lifestyle, and the everyday	

EMBRACING THE EXPERIENCE

Favorite Meals + Snacks	
Nervousness or Confidence	Hopes or Fears
Joy, Reverence + Awe	
Surprises	Changes
Complaints, Confessions, Heartaches, Challenges	

THE JOURNEY OF DISCOVERY

Learning, reading, listening to . . .	
How I connect with my partner	Focuses this month
Where I feel most loved and supported	
Advice	Reactions
Looking forward to . . .	

Three words to describe this time with baby:

_____

_____

This month in your life (a story to share or things to remember):

_____

_____

_____

_____

_____

_____

_____

_____

_____

_____

_____

_____

_____

Excitement, peace, and change at home: How has your new baby's presence shifted the energy in your family? What kind of effect has their arrival had on older siblings or your daily rhythm?

_____

_____

_____

_____

_____

Describe an average day in your life right now:

_____

_____

_____

_____

_____

_____

_____

_____

_____

_____

Look at all the ways your life has changed. How have your relationships shifted? What rituals or activities do you miss? What new rituals or activities do you love?

What are you enjoying about new motherhood? What's challenging or confusing?

_____

_____

_____

_____

_____

_____

_____

_____

_____

_____

_____

_____

_____

_____

_____

_____

_____

Take an inventory of how you're feeling physically, mentally, emotionally, and spiritually. Are there any areas in which you could use some extra support?

Do you feel you reliably have the time you need to replenish your Mother-well? Use this space to consider what kind of break would feel good to you (*i.e., uninterrupted time at home to read, meditate, nap, or take an unrushed shower, or time alone outside of the house to walk, take a class, be in nature, or go into town*), then experiment with trying them all out. Once you've found an activity or amount of alone time that allows you to feel satisfied and recharged, work with your partner to build this into your planned, regular schedule.

Look back at your journal entries from "Invite (Weeks 1–4)."
Which of this still resonates? How can you carry the most intrinsic
elements of *you* into motherhood?

Since these first entries, what have you learned? How do you see yourself differently? Sit for a moment to really be with the woman you are today.

about the author

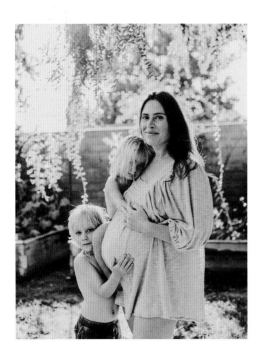

Rachel Garahan is a mother of three and personal-growth facilitator offering unconventional tools for self-discovery.

With an approach that is both easeful and effective, her journals, meditations, courses, and workshops empower individuals to reclaim space for themselves— to pause, find clarity, and tap into the answers within.

For playlists, recipes, bonus content and other resources, please visit *www.of-it-all.com/9-months-of-wonder.*

CONNECT ONLINE:

- WWW.OF-IT-ALL.COM
- @OF.IT.ALL

about familius

The most important work you ever do will be within the walls of your own home.

Familius is a global trade publishing company that publishes books and other content to help families be happy. To that end, we publish books for children and adults that invite families to live the Familius Ten Habits of Happy Families: *love together, play together, learn together, work together, talk together, heal together, read together, eat together, give together,* and *laugh together.*

VISIT OUR WEBSITE: WWW.FAMILIUS.COM